Bald n Dashing!

Hair Loss by Chance, Bald by Choice!

Cameron M. Clark

Bald n Dashing!

Hair Loss by Chance, Bald by Choice!

Cameron M. Clark

Bald n Dashing! Hair Loss by Chance, Bald by Choice!

Cameron M. Clark

Paul St. George Press © 2015

ISBN-13: 978-1534625389
ISBN-10: 1534625380

Disclaimer

Okay, let's get this out of the way…

I am not a medical doctor, so the following information in this book should not be seen as medical advice. The same goes for legal, financial, psychiatric, nutritional, fitness, mechanical and technological advice. The information in this book is purely for entertainment and discussion purposes only. If one chooses to adopt certain practices discussed in these pages, then they do so of their own choice and at their own risk.

Also, please note that there are a number of links in the footnotes to other websites citing my work. If you discover that a link is broken, please let me know at cameronmclark702@gmail.com.

Contents

Introduction

You're losing your hair.

So what?

Before you fire off a hate-riddled email to me, let me explain.

You've seen the television commercials, read the Internet ads and heard advertisements on the radio about hair restoration products or procedures. You've seen the ads for products that can 'cover' up or mask your balding spots with a spray or powder. There are tons of books and websites all over the Internet that are offering the latest cure for hair loss.

However, have you stopped to ask yourself what all of these advertising messages have in common?

They're all geared to make money by selling you a product that plays on emotions like fear, shame and regret. These companies want to sell you an idea that will ultimately lead to you buying their product and/or service. Their marketing people are everywhere and they want YOU to feel like crap so THEY can sell you a ton of product and make lots of money off of you.

So, in a way, congratulations!

I say 'congratulations,' because if you spent a few dollars on this book, you may have *chosen* to save thousands of dollars that you would have 'invested' in products and treatments that could lead to more problems and difficulty. By taking an hour to read this book, you may be saving yourself years of regret, embarrassment and frustration over adopting certain hair regrowth methods or hair restoration procedures that will just lead to more sadness and disappointment.

Now, you'll notice I'm not addressing the quality of any these products. Does a product that contains Minoxidil work? In some cases, yes. Do some of the pills on the market work in growing back a man's hair? Of course! Does a product that allows you to sprinkle or spray microscopic hairs onto the bare parts of your scalp fool the average human eye into thinking you have fuller, thicker hair? In many cases, yes.

But here's the problem: All of these scenarios and many others like it don't address the real problem.

The problem is that <u>you are insecure about your hair loss</u> and therefore, you might be insecure about other parts of your life.

My intent in writing this book isn't to delve into your psyche too deeply. It also isn't to explore all of your options for regrowing your hair or tricking your friends and family into thinking you have hair. Heck, this isn't even a book that takes some sort of neutral view toward that proposition. Instead, I wrote this book as a way of telling you that if you're losing your hair, whether your 18 or 48 years old, you should no longer feel shame about going bald.

I don't know you personally, so please don't take the above as some unfair judgment. However, I do know what it is like to lose my hair. Was I insecure about it? Yes! Of course! For quite a long time I was insecure about it, but something inside of me changed. My hope is that I can convey the secret of that change to you in the following pages.

As I prepared to write this book, I searched the Internet for resources that were similar to what I'd had in mind. I purchased a number of eBooks and other material that explored 'accepting' hair loss. Do you know what I found? I found that most of the books were apologetic or shameful in their tone. These were written like some weird 'self-confessional' transcript for a documentary or reality show and how the writer in question ultimately overcame the bummer of hair loss. On top of that, I found message boards all over the Internet, populated by men who were dealing with hair loss and not excited by it.

Well, I think it's time we get over the 'bummer of hair loss.' You want to be sad about losing your hair? Great, be sad. But after about 5 minutes of mourning and self-pity, embrace the NEW you. Your life goes on and do you know what? It gets better!

That's right! I said better! Not worse.

Too many of the books on Amazon and many Internet articles either convey a message that baldness is to be avoided at all costs or hidden from friends and family. There are also those who say that at best, if you go bald, life will move on and you should try to learn to cope with the new problem of hair loss. Cope?

I say screw all of that noise.

That's not what being Bald n Dashing is about! Losing your hair isn't a problem. Being Bald n Dashing is about taking a kick butt approach to your life and your relationships and saying 'yeah, I'm losing my hair. So what? You got a problem with that? Well, stop wasting my time!'

I'm not telling you go out and become a total jerk who treats others rudely. Instead, I'm saying it's time to be confident in your appearance. There are some practical things you can do to enhance those elements that make you who you are and show that you've moved past your hair loss. We're going to explore those in 'The 18 Actions to Take as a Bald Man.'

What do *you* want to get out of this book? After all, I wrote this book with one goal in mind: to tell you that becoming Bald n Dashing is one of the best 'bad' things that could ever happen to you. We'll be exploring the advantages to losing your hair in 'The 7 Benefits to Baldness.'

In the 'Case Studies' section, we explore the lives and careers of successful bald men from many walks of life. You will read about action stars, professional athletes, business leaders and others who chose to break up with their hair before it broke up with them. I've included photos of many of these Bald n Dashing men throughout the book.

It isn't okay that you're going bald; it's awesome that you're going bald!

The following pages aren't going to be the reassurances from someone who is in denial of his own hair loss. Believe me, I've dealt with all of those stages you go through in dealing with loss (the grief cycle, if you will) more than once. I never had to brainwash or convince myself into thinking that going bald was a good thing. I'm not delusional. Ever since I embraced my baldness in my late thirties, my life has improved immensely and I'll show you how you can improve yours.

Now join me on our journey to a better outlook on life and a better life in general as we work together for you to become 'Bald n Dashing!'

Preface

I like being bald.

I haven't always felt this way. It took some time.

In hindsight, I can't say I really ever looked that great with hair. However, I looked worse when it was thinning and then I looked almost as bad when I tried hiding the fact I was losing my hair.

The genesis for this book and its message came to me a while ago, but I chose not to act on it at first. The project kept calling to me repeatedly and I refused to heed its siren call. Eventually, I gave in and this book, 'Bald n Dashing! Hair Loss by Chance, Bald by Choice!' is the result of my wearing down.

After completing the three books I'd intended to finish in 'The Great Big Quote Books' series, I had considered this book as my next project. However, before beginning this project, I searched the market to see if there was something out there that reflected what I'd been feeling: A book that took a bold, yet humorous look at going bald and losing your hair. Nothing reached out and grabbed my attention.

Sure, there were humorous books about going bald with funny-looking covers that talked about being confident in general with the prospect of choosing to be bald. But they were mostly apologetic in their approach. Many read like confessional essays. There was still this sense of grief attached to the idea that hair loss made the reader feel like an inferior human being and that this was something to be mourned over. There were books about taking the steps of grieving your hair loss as though your beloved grandmother or favorite uncle had just passed away. After seeing books with this apologetic tone, I'd had enough.

Then there were the books on Amazon and other websites that purported to have the 'cures' to hair loss. They covered the theories of hair loss and the 'remedies' available. Preying on the fear, weakness, desperation and insecurity of balding men (and some balding women), many of these guides appeared to be the same recycled ideas that were likely being recommended by the traveling snake oil salesman a century and a half ago. Some covers would show women with luscious, thick hair that was obviously supposed to incite a jealousy in the potential reader leading to an impulse buy. The majority of covers available showed an insecure-looking man with either thinning hair or a baldhead looking into the mirror with a sad look on his face while holding a comb.

Here's a quick example. The cover below is the original cover that my well-meaning regular cover designer sent me after I'd specifically asked for a cover that showed a bald man for what he really could be: attractive, confident and capable.

Instead, she sent me a cover design showing an unattractive, anonymous bald man with his head in his hands.

See the problem?

She was so used to getting cover orders for books dealing with hair loss and going bald that this was what automatically came to her mind, despite my instructions. There are so many books and messages saying the same thing to men who are losing their hair: be ashamed to be bald.

It is time to take a stand.

There is no shame in going bald. Say it with me, 'There is no shame in losing my hair.' Louder now! 'THERE IS NO SHAME IN LOSING MY HAIR!' Ok, people are starting to look. That's good enough.

I'm not going to argue whether the 21st Century has caused men and women to become the most-enlightened in the Earth's history, but the thing I think most of us can all appreciate is that the ideas of 'tolerance' and 'acceptance' seem to be more widespread in western society than they ever have been. Is there still a stigma against balding men? In some corners of society, there are likely a few people who feel that way. But we're not worried about them. Our lives go on, their lives continue and they have to live with their superficial and sometimes prejudicial attitudes.

Sure, our society has a long way to go, but compared to 50, 60 or even 100 years ago, there really are very few things you can do to your image or appearance that would be perceived as 'counter cultural' or rebellious.

Will we share laughs in the following pages? I hope so. Will there be tears as well? Maybe, but I hope not. All of the tears you've shed over your hair loss should be in the past. My hope is that this book will give you the desire to embrace the 'new' you without shame or embarrassment.

Be Bald by Choice!
Be Bald n Dashing!

Cameron Clark
June 2015

P.S. - I hired a different designer for the below covers. They modeled what I had in mind all along for the 'Bald n Dashing' man!

Acknowledgements

I just want to give a quick shout out to my daughter, Brinley for giving me the idea for the subtitle of this book. Such a simple, yet to-the-point statement: Hair loss by chance, bald by choice! Thanks, Brinnie!

Also, thank you to my two other wonderful children for loving their dad and supporting him in the writing of this book.

A big thank you to my wife, the only editor I can afford. I love you and appreciate the years of support you've given me as I've worked on my many writing projects.

Thank you to my friends and family who have always accepted me for who I am. I've learned more from many of you than you will ever learn from me.

Also, a quick thank you to Paul St. George Press for their continual belief and support in me to make these books ready for publishing.

Finally, I want to dedicate this book to the men (and some of the women) who were way ahead of me in choosing the Bald n Dashing look. You have blazed a trail that I can appreciate and I hope others will take courage from your example.

7 Facts

Before we get into the specifics of your choosing to start this new phase of your life, we should get a few things out of the way. The following are just a few thoughts I've had which seem to apply to most people as they deal with hair loss.

First fact: You are not your hair and your hair is not you.

I'm not the first person to put that message into the world. There are many out there before me who have stated this in print and in other places. The difference is that I might be the first to tell you this unapologetically.

In other words, if you are a nice person on the inside and treat other people with respect, it has nothing to do with your hair or lack of hair. If you're a mean person or a jerk, you probably have some work to do on yourself from the inside to become a better person. However, none of this is other people's fault. Nor is it the fault of your hair follicles.

Second fact: There are things you can to do to either draw attention away from your baldhead or if you want, you can draw attention toward it. Draw attention to it? I know that sounds crazy to some people, but there are definitely situations where this might work to your advantage. Hopefully, by the end of this book, you'll see what I'm talking about.

Third fact: Bald has come a long way.

While it is true that when a Hollywood starlet shaves her head for a role (or before a possible drug test), she still attracts the attention of the paparazzi and the general public. A man, on the other hand, who is bald by choice usually gets less attention than he did even 20 or 30 years ago. Think about it, Yul Brynner, Telly Savalas and a select few 'Hollywood tough guys' would put the razor to their heads and then suddenly, it became 'The Yul Brynner look' or 'The Telly Savalas.' People didn't know what else to call it back then, because it was so rare.

Now, actors, athletes and other well-known public figures have adopted this look in varying degrees and the press rarely makes mention of it.

Fourth fact: If you're insecure about your thinning hair or all of the parts of scalp that are showing, it will become apparent to those around you that you are feeling insecure and they will treat you accordingly. A lack of confidence is a very real thing and it is up to you to develop the confidence necessary to show you couldn't care less that you're losing your hair. Keep reading. I have some ideas that may help.

Fifth fact: Studies have found that men who choose to break up with their hair before their hair breaks up with them (bald by choice) are perceived as more masculine and therefore, more physically dominant than their follically-gifted counterparts. Yes, many of the articles and studies will tell you that the trade-off is that you may appear less attractive than men with hair. However, the studies cannot quantify *how* much less attractive. After all, there are many sane and normal women out there who are drawn to men with no hair. Not as a fetish, but because they really find that look attractive.

Sixth fact: When you decide to shave your hair off, you will need to adopt certain practices to maintain the health of the skin on your scalp. This book will cover some of those things so you can avoid the problems attached to developing a rash, razor burn or sunburn.

Seventh fact: The terms 'buzzed' and 'shaved' are used frequently in this book.

What's not so clear at first is which term applies to which. In a general sense, I will use these terms interchangeably in this book. However, I believe a 'buzzed' head is one where an electric device like clippers has trimmed the hair and there is still a short length of hair that is visible on the scalp. A 'shaved' head is one that has had a razor blade taken to it and gotten as close to the scalp as possible. Generally, the shaved head has no visible hair left on it for around 24 hours.

There are many other facts that we could cite here, but I think we've established that there are some things that will work to your advantage as you adopt the Bald n Dashing lifestyle and there are some things of which you should continue to be aware.

My Story: Confessions of a Balding Man

What you are about to read is a brief narrative of my own experience with hair loss. Before I buzzed my head, there were moments of anxiety over the prospect of losing my hair. However, I have yet to regret my ultimate decision to 'break up' with my hair before it all broke up with me.

The Revelation

I still remember where I was sitting when I found out I was losing my hair.

It was in the utility room of my parents' house adjacent to the garage. I was eighteen-and-a-half years old.

My sister, a trained cosmetologist, was cutting my hair after my being away from home to college for two semesters. During high school, Cassell would cut my hair every six weeks or so. At the time, I still had a decent head of hair that I usually wore in a pompadour hairstyle by sweeping my blonde locks to the side. It was an easy haircut to maintain.

After I'd been gone to college for about 10 months, my sister's memory of my hairline was still vivid enough that the moment she began wetting my hair down for the cut, she told me I was going bald. I laughed at first thinking it was a joke. However, when she said she wasn't joking, my mood turned sour. I hadn't even reached the age of 21 and already my hair was giving up the ghost. Cassell said it was receding, but just a little at a time. She gave me no prognosis as to when it would all fall out. In hindsight, how could she have known? After all, I was just a young man and already nature was taking one of my outward signs of virility and vitality, one strand at a time.

As I got older, I didn't think about it too much. I suppose it might have been a mix of ignorance and denial. After all, I was doing all of the fun things that young men in their late teens do. I didn't even give it any thought that girls my age might notice that I was losing my hair.

The Realization

It wasn't until I was serving a religious mission for my church at the age of twenty that I had the first real encounter with the prospect of going bald. I'd been serving in this voluntary capacity for just over a year when I was eating dinner at the home of a church member. His wife asked me point blank how old I was. Instead of answering, I asked her why she would ask that. She said she just wondered how old a man could be to still serve a mission. Using charm, I deflected her question and asked her how old I looked. I expected a guess of 23 or 24 at most. Instead, she guessed that I was around 27 or 28 years old and then observed that it might have been because I was losing my hair.

I'm sure I turned three shades of red that night. What a thing to say! Even to this day, I'm a little surprised at the audacity she had to continue discussing such an awkward topic when clearly I was not comfortable discussing it at length. Regardless, I smiled back at her and told her I had just turned 20 years old a couple months earlier.

The 'Kit'

Near the end of my mission, the hair loss must have been getting more noticeable in the pictures I sent home to my mom. Before the next Christmas, Cassell had sent me a 'kit' of products that were supposed to 'thicken' my hair. This kit included 'thickening' shampoo, 'thickening' conditioner, some sort of 'stimulating' spray and a miniature 'strainer' that I could place over the shower drain so I could actually count how many hairs were falling out of my head.

Whoever wrote the marketing copy for these products was very careful not to promise that new hair was going to grow back. However, these wordsmith geniuses were so convincing in their copy that I wore down and put my hope and trust in these strange products. Maybe I was so tired of the thought of going bald, that I really believed using these chemicals and applying them to my scalp morning and night would grow back my hair. Instead, it turned my scalp red for a few minutes and then my scalp would return to a normal color. Supposedly the spray was designed to increase the blood flow to my hair follicles and that would lead to me growing back my hair.

The Powder

Years later, I was living in Las Vegas. I'd been married to the girl of my dreams for many years and had been keeping my hair quite short for just about as long of a time.

It was shortly after I'd moved to Las Vegas that a close relative introduced me to a product that changed the way I looked at myself for years to come. It was a powder of synthetic fibers that were statically charged to stick to my existing hair and scalp. These tiny fibers created the illusion that I had a full head of thick hair. I was 29 years old at the time and already a noticeable thin spot was coming through the crown of my head. It was a few inches wide and was starting to show up in pictures. Oy! It was time to take drastic action.

Morning, noon and night, I would sprinkle this powder on my head before going out in public anywhere. I would do it before going to work, the gym, church or even a quick trip to the grocery store. I would even keep a small travel-sized container in my car for touch ups when it rained or if I bumped my head on the inside of the car's roof.

I started with the medium brown, but noticed it gave off a reddish tint under artificial light. I switched to dark brown which was much harder to detect. I did have encounters with someone who may not have been well-versed in the art of social discretion. She told me that my hair looked like I dyed it purple. I just sheepishly grinned and made up some silly joke to cover up the secret and hide my insecurity. At the time, I would have rather had her think that I was dying the gray out of my hair, but that I still had a nearly full head of hair than to think I was going bald and trying to cover it up.

In hindsight, I now realize I'd been developing a bit of a mental dependence on this product. It worked rather well, but I couldn't stand the thought of leaving the house without it on my scalp.

The Revolution

After some of these 'critical' conversations I'd been having, it was becoming more and more apparent to me that I was not fooling as many people as I had a few years earlier, or maybe I'd thought I was fooling them all along. Regardless, I was facing a crucial decision.

A couple of events occurred within a matter of weeks that ultimately led me to decide to buzz my hair off. A friend of mine at church asked me why my hair was giving off a purplish tint. It was after some cajoling that he finally had gotten my secret out of me. He was in his early 20s, so subtlety was not one of his stronger qualities.

'Are you vain?' he asked.

'No,' I said.

'Then why are you so worried about people finding out you're going bald?'

I had no answer. I just thought a lot about it and mulled that statement over in my head again and again.

The second event that came about the same time was that I was to be one of the youth supervisors at my oldest daughter's church youth camp in the middle of summer. It was at a dude ranch in central Utah and was going to last around 4 or 5 days. The activities at this camp being both outdoor and indoor would require the wearing and removing of my hat several times throughout the day. I played out in my mind all of the potential scenarios of how I could make the powder work for me while in those close quarters with other adult leaders nearby and sitting across from me.

I thought of the powder smearing down my forehead in a mix of sweat and dirt. It would be noticeable in the open light to whomever I was facing. There was only going to be so many times I could say that I had some dirt on my forehead. I also thought of how the inside of my hats would be colored brown. On top of that, I thought of all of the potential 'holes' the powder would leave in my hair allowing my scalp to show through.

Every scenario I ran through in my mind resulted in the potential for embarrassment and long-winded explanations. It was then that I started to realize I really was being insecure about my baldness and that for some reason, I'd been holding on to some bizarre shame for losing my hair through natural causes. My friend was right. Had I developed some dependence on this product?

The decision wasn't made overnight. It took me a few more days to come to terms with something I'd been deceiving myself about for nearly two decades! I was going bald. Were there remedies like minoxidil and finasteride? Sure, but this late in the game that wasn't going to grow in nearly enough hair to cover my scalp in time for girls camp. Not to mention that the listed potential side effects of those drugs had always kept me away from ever purchasing them in the first place. Why start now?

So, the night before we left for the camp, I went to a local hair salon that specialized in 'clipping' hair off and had them buzz it all off with a #1 guard. It was liberating.

The Result?

I returned home later that night from the hair salon and received a very positive response from my wife.

'It draws my eyes to your eyes,' she said immediately.

I played it cool as I thought she was just flattering me.

'Also, it seems to make your nose appear a bit smaller.'

I was willing to take as a positive that too. Not that I'd had a big nose in the first place, but it sounded like a positive.

My kids weren't as big of fans at first, but my oldest daughter started rubbing my head 'for luck.'

At the camp, no one really said anything, though I'm sure most of them noticed that all of a sudden at the top of my buzzed head, there were a few bald patches where it had appeared previously that I'd grown hair. The best part? I could take off my hat anytime.

Since that time, I have buzzed my head at least once a week with no guard on the clippers. Could I go shorter and just shave my head with an actual razor and shaving cream? Sure, but I like this look right now. I don't care that it is clear that I have bald patches. It is something that I wear with a measure of confidence now. I think that comes through to the people with whom I meet.

I am bald by choice and I don't care who knows it.

That's what being Bald n Dashing is all about!

A Brief History of Baldness

O Captain! My Captain!

To understand baldness in all its forms, we need to go way back!

Way, way back to 1987, when a new television series hit the screens. This wasn't just any television series though, this was a show spun off of its super successful predecessor *Star Trek*. The new series was going to be called *Star Trek: The Next Generation*.

Set a century after the era where Captain James T. Kirk helmed the USS Enterprise on a 5-year exploratory mission, this was a show that was going to go into the further realms of space to seek out new life and new civilizations. It was a show of hope and optimism. A show with a sexy new cast that more accurately reflected the racial and sexual diversity of our current society along with an alien or two to make things interesting. It was a show not only about tolerance, but acceptance of the fact we are not all the same, but rather unique and special in our own —.

Waitaminnit! What was this?

A bald captain at the helm of the new Starship Enterprise? Could this be? A BALD man? Surely the producers were legally blind or medically declared insane to allow a man with a balding pate to lead this band of star rovers.

But it was not a mistake. Shakespearean actor Patrick Stewart was the choice of the producers. He had won them over with his confidence and gravitas on the stage. Soon, Stewart would become a favorite for many fans of the show, young and old.

However, Stewart didn't just waltz onto the set, audition for the now-iconic role of Captain Jean-Luc Picard and take the part. No, Star Trek historians tell a different tale.

As the story goes, original series creator and executive producer on the new series, Gene Roddenberry initially was against casting Stewart as Picard. Roddenberry was open about his desire to cast a younger captain with a full head of hair. And could you blame him? After all, William Shatner had defined what a starship captain was all about with his swashbuckling approach to Captain James T. Kirk. And full head of hair... or rather, almost full head of hair.

It is believed that Shatner had been losing his hair even as the original *Star Trek* series had been in production and at some point began wearing hairpieces to cover the appearance of hair loss.[1]

Though Roddenberry resisted, Stewart had an ally in his corner: producer Robert H. Justman, who had been impressed with Stewart's audition for the role. Roddenberry didn't give up until they'd exhausted their search for another actor to play the starship captain and finally relented in giving Stewart the role. Talk about starting off on the wrong foot.

After winning over Roddenberry, Justman and Stewart had to win over the executives at Paramount, as they were the main corporate arm responsible for distribution of the show. At the suggestion of the producers, Stewart wore a hairpiece at the first meeting with the Paramount executives. I'm not sure what was said during the meeting, but one thing that came out it was that the Paramount executives said he had the

---

[1] An Internet search will reveal many articles about theories as to what kind of hairpieces Shatner wore during his days on 'Star Trek: The Original Series.' This one goes meta and talks about those sites:

http://www.deseretnews.com/article/865578034/Shatners-toupee-is-a-hair-raising-pastime.html?pg=all job as long as he didn't wear that 'ridiculous' hair piece.[2]

Roddenberry's prejudice against Stewart along with the producers' fear of intolerance was unfounded as *Star Trek: The Next Generation* became the first and only syndicated series to be nominated for an Emmy Award for Best Dramatic Series. It received 18 Emmy awards and a large number of accolades from the science fiction community. With his somewhat brooding and serious, yet undeniably Bald n Dashing approach to the character, Patrick Stewart became a household name and started a legacy of 'bald is beautiful' awareness for years to come.

The Real History of Baldness

Ok, you got me.

Baldness didn't start with a television show. Baldness has likely been around from the beginning of mankind. Whether you believe that Adam and Eve were the first humans on the planet or you believe it was that guy who came out of Africa 90 000 years

---

[2] Check out awesome fact number 4:

http://moviepilot.com/posts/2014/12/22/8-awesome-facts-about-star-trek-the-next-generation-2535675?lt_source=external,manual ago who is our ancestral forefather or something else, there was likely always a bald guy (or sometimes a bald girl) in the social group. After all, the Bible says Adam lived to well past 900 years of age. You don't think he lost a few hairs along the way?

Moving along down the corridors of time, it is rather well known among historians that baldness and hair loss along with the accompanying search for a cure was a focus for some of the Egyptians as many historians point to 'The Ebers Papyrus' as the source of the cure. The cure was said to have included fats extracted from a lion, hippopotamus, crocodile and other animals. Sounds simple enough, right?[3]

A bit later in history, one of the first well-known personal accounts of baldness can be found in the Book of Kings regarding the prophet Elisha. A few of the local youth were mocking Elisha saying 'Go up, thou baldhead; Go up, thou baldhead.'[4] How did he get the kids to leave him alone? Well, the Bible doesn't say he had anything to do with it directly, but female bears to came out of the

---

[3] http://www.history.com/news/history-lists/9-bizarre-baldness-cures

[4] 2 Kings 2:23 (King James Version)

forest and attacked those ignorant kids. I suppose that's one way to solve the problem.

Though it had been around for ceremonious occasions in numerous cultures for centuries, the laurel wreath became a part of Roman Emperor Julius Caesar's image. When growing the back part of his hair long and then combing it forward over the top of his baldhead (the ancient version of a combover), he became desperate for other remedies. Ultimately, Caesar wore the laurel wreath around the crown part of his head to serve as a type of toupee. There are many who believe Caesar was full on bald and this was a way of masking his insecurity.[5]

Fast-forward a millennia and a half to the 16th and 17th Centuries in Europe when the wig was introduced. Many men in the higher classes had taken to the wearing of wigs as a symbol of their status and class. Kings, magistrates, lawyers and many others in high society would don a different wig as a part of their entire ensemble. There were also military units in Europe during this time that thought outfitting officers with wigs was a good idea. The stigma of hair loss was still prevalent in many older societies and followed

---

[5]   http://www.history.com/news/from-hippo-fat-to-vacuum-helmets-a-history-of-baldness-prevention

down through the ages to this more 'enlightened' society.[6] Having hair, even during that time, was an outward sign of youth and virility.

Ahhhhh, some old myths are hard to kill.

As western society headed into the 19th Century, baldness had still not been 'cured.' However, that did not stop many men and some women from concocting 'remedies' that were supposed to suppress, stop or even reverse hair loss. As has been said by an old showman, there's a sucker born every minute and balding men were not immune.

The snake oil salesmen and women have gotten much more clever in the 21st Century. An Internet search for the many hokey remedies and solutions to hair loss will reveal a theory that hats were causing hair loss. Another was that regular shampooing of the scalp would cause hair to fall out faster. Yet another myth that still lasts to this day was that the gene for baldness was passed down through the mother. Of course, these false beliefs along with the many 'remedies' that accompanied them proved to be false.

---

[6]

http://en.wikipedia.org/wiki/Wig#16th_and_17th_centuries

More importantly they represented a bigger problem: That baldness was some *problem* that had to be *cured*.

Where the Real Problems Began

Personally, I lament the gullibility of those insecure men in past generations, who parted with many hard-earned dollars in the hopes that the 'snake-oil' they rubbed into their scalp would ultimately grow even just a few strands of hair on top of their heads. Now it seems, that this gullibility has transformed into full-blown desperation thanks to the many advertisements targeting men with the idea of hair replacement surgery.

We've all seen the many ads of the actor with a sad expression on his face as he looks into the mirror at his thinning hair and tries to comb it this way and that. Accompany those images with a smooth-talking voice-over guy telling you how the world is judging him for his hair loss.

What comes next?

Instant customers.

In earlier drafts of this book, I wrote an extensive history on the hair transplant. After much thought, I didn't see how it would benefit you, the reader. My message is one of courage and hope. Why give another moment's credence to the businessmen and women who would just love for you to sign over your scalp for them to cut up for a low five figure sum?

I met a friend at lunch other other day. He is almost completely bald on top of his head and has chosen to shave the rest of the hair extremely short. He told me that he'd just received a LinkedIn message from some enterprising doctor in Los Angeles who was trolling the LinkedIn profiles to solicit business. Talk about desperate and opportunistic. This guy was merely preying on my friend's insecurities. He laughed at the solicitation and deleted it.

Think about it.

There is so much money to be made off of men (and some women) who are losing their hair.

When a car company runs an ad on television, do they do it from the standpoint that you are already satisfied with your current car?

In other words, does the script go like this?

We know your 2011 car is a sweet ride and it still has all of the things you need to get from point A to point B. However, you might be interested in something that we have new on the market. This vehicle has a lot of new features, but a lot of the same features as what you already have. You know, on second thought, take it or leave it. It's a great car though.'

No, the script goes more like this:

'Your current car is a piece of junk! No one takes you seriously in that thing. You think you're a self-respecting man in that 2011 vehicle? That thing doesn't even have wireless hookups. So inadequate. So lame. Not only are you unattractive to women, even your own family members don't respect you for your choice to drive that old car. So pathetic.'

Okay. The second script was way over-the-top, but how aren't those the same marketing techniques the hair restoration companies run?

Again, the advertisements usually start out with a guy looking into the mirror with a worried look on his face as the voiceover man asks the question 'Are you worried that your hair is falling out?' The sad, balding man then looks into the mirror at the camera and nods and we're off to the races. What follows are actors and actresses in lab coats talking to the man and reassuring him that even though it feels like it's the end of the world because of his hair loss, it's not. Yes, if you put an actor or actress in a lab coat, all of a sudden they become credible.

We've all seen it. It's silly and it's manipulative.

Now that we've briefly explored many facets of the history of baldness, let's take a look at some real life cases of men who chose the Bald n Dashing look for themselves.

Case Studies

I want to explore the lives of some of the men who set the standard in becoming Bald by Choice. These men said to the world, 'Yeah, I'm bald. So what? I've got a lot more to offer you than the hair that is or isn't on my head.'

We already discussed Patrick Stewart, but there are many who came before and many more who have come after this iconic actor's foray into fame as a starship captain. My goal in shining the spotlight on a number of these men is to show you that no matter who you are or what your physical make up, it is likely there is a balding 'role model' out there for you.

And now in no particular order:

Yul Brynner

Brynner was likely not the first actor to maintain a shaved head during much of his career, but he was one of the more famous and well-known for his time. In 1951, Brynner shaved his head for his role as the King of Siam in the London and Broadway musical 'The King and I' and he never looked back. In fact, this distinctive look was likely what led the famed film director Cecil B.

Demille to choose the Russian actor for the role of Rameses II in the 1956 blockbuster movie 'The Ten Commandments.'

Was Brynner going bald when he shaved his hair off for 'The King and I?'

Does it matter?

While Brynner wore a wig for some of the roles he played from time to time, he maintained the shaved head appearance until his death in 1985. He was not only an accomplished and award-winning stage and film actor, Brynner was also a prolific photographer, author and accomplished guitarist.

Why did he accomplish so much?

Maybe its because he didn't have to waste time worrying about his hair.

Bruce Willis

Born on a US military base in West Germany and raised in New Jersey, Willis might have seemed like just any other guy. However, during his career, his films have grossed well in excess of $3 billion USD at the time of this writing.[7]

---

[7]
http://www.boxofficemojo.com/people/chart/?view=Actor&sort=gross&order=DESC&id=brucewillis.htm

Willis first rose to prominence starring in the mid-80s television hit 'Moonlighting.' He took a turn as the ultimate 'everyman' New York City cop in one of the coolest action movies of all time: 'Die Hard.'

It was no secret that Willis's hairline was receding by the time he'd appeared in the first 'Die Hard.' That didn't stop him though. The man continued to rake in hundreds of millions of dollars at the box office by appearing in movies like the 'Die Hard' sequels, 'Twelve Monkeys,' 'The Fifth Element,' 'The Sixth Sense,' 'Armageddon' and 'Unbreakable.'

Willis's hair line has changed over the years for the roles he's had to play in various films due to the wigs and other hair pieces he has worn. However, when the man goes out in public, he doesn't worry about the fact he's showing scalp. Sure, from time-to-time, he is photographed wearing a funky hat, but for the most part, he is a confident dude.

I remember reading an article a couple years ago where his daughter Rumor tells of struggling with what kind of hairstyle to wear next. He suggested that she could just shave it off. That would save her some time. An action star and a comedian!

Michael Jordan

I defy any kid who grew up in the 80s to find a guy who was cooler than basketball legend, Michael Jordan. Taking a look at pictures of him in the height of his basketball career and even now, the man still looks young, energetic and vibrant. I think part of that has to do with the fact that he started shaving his head so long ago.

Jordan is a giant among many of the basketball greats in the history of the game and he hasn't slowed down into retirement. Jordan has shown that you can look better without hair. I mean after all these years in the spotlight sans hair, don't those earlier pictures of Michael Jordan with hair almost look awkward and out of place?

Sean Connery

This Scotsman was the original 007. Tall, dark, handsome… and balding. With the exception of John Wayne was there a movie star manlier than Connery in 1960s cinema? I doubt it. A former bodybuilding competitor and model in the late 1950s, Connery went on to define one of the most iconic movie roles in the 20th Century: Bond, James Bond.

As he progressed through his film career as the debonair super spy, Connery was a casanova with the ladies and was usually the first to break up with them in their short-lived romances. However, one breakup he accomplished before he could be dumped was with his hair. Connery embraced the baldness and took new cues for acting roles that still brought forth the manly aspect of his character. He did wear a hairpiece in such blockbuster films as 'The Rock' and 'The Hunt for Red October.' However, he was a sex symbol to people all around the world even heading into the 1990s and isn't ashamed to go out into public bald.

Samuel L. Jackson

An iconic actor of the late 20th-Century, Jackson had played everything from a hostage negotiator gone rogue to an FBI agent trapped on a plane with thousands of snakes along with a number of other awesome roles. However, Jackson's star rose to a whole new level of fame appearing as Colonel Nicholas J. Fury, the head of S.H.I.E.L.D. in a series of Marvel movies that included the 2012 blockbuster 'The Avengers.'

Though he was well over 60 years old in that film, Jackson was able to pull off an energetic, much younger look, in part because of his decidedly bald pate. A little known fact is that when Marvel Comics was updating their comic book universe with what they called the 'ultimate' version, the creative team that oversaw the creation of the modern Avengers modeled their new design of Colonel Fury after the iconic actor.[8] This was years before anyone had even thought of an Avengers movie! Can you think of a more complimentary homage to your reputation than that?

Anderson Silva

Considered by many (including myself) to be the greatest mixed martial artist of all time, this Brazilian holds the record for the longest title defense streak in the middleweight division of the UFC.[9] I have been a fan of mixed martial arts competition for many years and I can tell you that in all of the fights I've ever watched, Silva's have been some of the most entertaining. There have been a few stinkers in there as well, but overall, he is a fighter whose combination of grace, style and power is unsurpassed. While his career fizzled in recent years due to a string of losses and

---

[8]

http://en.wikipedia.org/wiki/Ultimate_Nick_Fury#Publication_history

[9] At the time of this writing (2015).

unimpressive victories, Silva was always a force to be reckoned with.

I can't recall ever seeing a picture or video clip of Silva with hair. He cuts it as close to the scalp as he can. He's a good-looking guy too; just ask my wife.

Dwayne 'The Rock' Johnson

After Hulk Hogan, is there another professional wrestler with more charisma, more popularity and name recognition and more outward confidence than 'The Rock?' I have a hard time thinking there is. Yes, he started his wrestling career with a decent head of hair, but as the years wore on, the writing was on the wall; Johnson's hair line was receding.

So he did what any confident fellow would do in his situation and he became bald by choice. This has led to a meteoric rise in fame as one of Hollywood's premiere action stars.

Jack Welch

When I was putting this book together, I didn't want to just focus on athletes, actors and musicians. I thought it was important to shine a spotlight that would reflect off of the baldheads of men who've succeeded in other walks of life. One of the most outwardly successful has been former General Electric CEO Jack Welch. He also may stand out from this list as a man who is clearly bald on top, but has kept a little bit of side and back hair. I think he'd benefit from a complete shave, but I don't have an estimated net worth of over $700 million.

Here is a man who is credited with increasing the value of GE by 4000% during his tenure. Many say he was a hard-driving executive, but many would have to agree that he did get things done. Shorter in stature than the average American male in height at 5'7", Welch is the kind of man who was determined to succeed and he did.

Vin Diesel

A Hollywood success story about persistence and perseverance, Diesel actually had gone to Hollywood to make it as an actor in the early 1990s. Like nearly every performer trying to make their way up the ladder of success, he struggled. At some point, Diesel moved back to live with his parents in New York. While there, he learned about how he could take control of his career and future by making his own films.

When he returned to Hollywood, Diesel had settled on the look we all know and attach to him today. He seems to do best in the action star roles and doesn't show any signs of slowing down.

Chris Daughtry

Whether you like his mainstream rock sound or not, you have to admit that Daughtry stands out in a business that still thinks that 'boy bands' with hair are a safe bet. Since before he was a contestant on fifth season of the television show 'American Idol,' Daughtry's shaved head shouted to the judges, the public and anyone else who was watching that he was marching to the beat of his own drum. His earlier than expected departure from the show became the lynchpin for his success as one of the greatest success stories to come out of the entire series.

Daughtry has gone on to be a best-selling recording artist over and over again and will likely continue as a successful musician in the years to come.

Jason Statham

While he hasn't shorn his hair down to the scalp, Statham has defined a unique look in our society that had been around prior to him popularizing it. However, it feels like he's made it his own. Square-jawed and usually lean and muscular on camera, Statham has portrayed many characters who are proficient in martial arts fighting and other skills.

When I was compiling this list, I almost put Statham at the top because he truly does represent the message I'm trying to get across: 'I'm going bald, so what? You don't like it? Well, screw you.' He does it so well by the fact that he allows some hair to grow in at the sides and the back. He's also sporting a five o'clock shadow much of the time. It also hasn't hurt him with the ladies.

There's no doubt he's been losing his hair for many years going back to his first appearances in movies like 'Snatch' and 'Lock, Stock and Two Smoking Barrels,' but he's never let that stop him. If anything, the best may still be yet to come with this action hero.

Stephen R. Covey

Whether you believe in the power of self-help or not, the late Dr. Covey was a man who stood (bald) head and shoulders above the rest during his lifetime. You may remember him best for writing the book 'The 7 Habits of Highly Effective People,' though he wrote many other business bestsellers that are still used today.

A scholar and an entrepreneur, Covey was the real deal. He was asked to meet with world leaders like President Bill Clinton to discuss his ideas on leadership and organizational management. If you were looking for a bald role model who exuded the confidence of a man who didn't care that he was losing his hair, I think you'd be safe with Covey, who was shaving his head going back to the 80s.

Andre Agassi

A world-famous, top-ranked championship tennis player, Agassi drew much attention for his long locks and aggressive playing style on the court in the 1980s. For years, he was considered a sex symbol in tennis with his fit physique and good looks.

At some point though, the hair had to go. And off it all went, never to return. Again, Agassi drew the eyes of the world to him. He was unapologetic about shaving off his hair and he appears to have never looked back. Agassi has gone on to be a prominent figure in philanthropy, particularly in the Las Vegas community.

Matt Lauer

Matt Lauer has been hosting national news programs for more than two decades. Naturally, he was going to age in front of the camera. As he has aged, Lauer faced the prospect of hair loss. There were rumors and even some photographic evidence that Lauer may have used the hair powder product I'd used to cover up his bald spots. At some point, Lauer realized it was better to just embrace the bald look.

Those are just a few case studies that have hopefully helped you see that no matter what life has dealt you, you too can be a success. You'll notice that these men come in all shapes and sizes, economic and cultural backgrounds and yet the one thing they have in common is that they didn't let losing their hair get in the way of the bigger picture.

That's what I've been wanting for you too!

Keep reading! What follows are a few advantages to being bald.

The 7 Benefits to Baldness

There are probably dozens, if not hundreds of benefits to being bald, but I'm going to highlight a few that are usually the most common among balding men:

1. Save Time and Money

This one is a serious no-brainer. After all, if you have no or little hair, you won't be spending money and time on shampoos, hair conditioning products, styling gels and more. On top of that, if you embrace the 'bald by choice' mentality, you will no longer be susceptible to the many 'hair loss solutions' like the drugs and pills on the market. Further, you will no longer consider getting a second mortgage on your house to pay for that hair transplant that may or may not work out fully for you. Much of this is covered in the next chapter.

2. No More Primping After Stepping out of Inclement Weather

When I had hair, I always felt a little funny going into inclement weather. Add to it that I needed to check my hair after getting out of the wind or rain. The same goes for taking off a hat.

Well, not anymore!

I have always felt that it seemed vain and a little less masculine for a man to be worried about how his hair looked after he came in from the outside. At the same time, if it was now all sticking up in the back or if one side stuck out way too far, then that looks kind of stupid too.

The solution?

Just shave or buzz it all down to next to nothing. Problem solved.

3. Bald Looks Good with Just about Anything

Some people will disagree with me on this next point and that's fine. When you think of looking at pictures from 10 or 20 years ago, other than the clothes, what is the other dead giveaway? The hairstyles you wore at the time, of course. Take away that remaining amount of hair and you don't have to worry about dating yourself in pictures. Well, at least your hair won't give you away; fashion trends may be another story.

Whether it's a suit, a tuxedo or just a plain old button down shirt and jeans, the bald guy can pull it all off without much thought. On top of that, whether you have a slim build, carry around some muscle or you're working on losing that spare tire, a shaved or buzzed head will go really well with your look.

4. One Way of Showing You've Overcome One of the 7 Deadly Sins

This might be a bit idealistic and to some, it might seem a bit spiritual or moral to others. After all, vanity has to do with more than just our hair. It is possible to be vain about a thousand other things without our hair getting in the way. The good news is just like in Benefit # 1, there will be no primping and preening in front of a mirror when coming out of a situation that is less than congenial to your hair.

When I pondered my reasons for considering the buzzing off of my hair, this one kept coming back to me. In many ways, I still fight with vanity. However, after much thought, I realized that holding on to the remaining hair I had and using a powder to cover up the bald spots daily just seemed more vain to me.

This conquering of vanity leads me to the next point.

5. Women Appreciate Confidence over Vanity

In my experience, vanity is not an attractive quality to most women. Imagine what a woman might be thinking if you spend more than a couple minutes fixing your hair.

Am I saying that you shouldn't care at all about your outward appearance or that you shouldn't take care of yourself? Not at all! In fact, because you are losing your hair and may be choosing to become bald by choice, it is best that you maintain an outwardly competent and confident appearance and that you show you can take care of yourself.

There have been studies done in recent years citing the fact that bald men are seen as more masculine.[10] The same study says that some women find men without hair to be less attractive than men with hair, but that same man is considered more dominant. Remember, this is for men who have chosen to shave off their hair.

So if perception were reality in some cases, how would you rather be perceived?

There will still be superficial women out there after you shave your head, just like there are superficial men who say they're only attracted to women with a certain hair color or body type. It's not up to you to try to control the way other people think. Just

---

[10]   http://healthland.time.com/2012/09/28/shave-it-off-how-bald-guys-can-look-more-manly-and-dominant/

know that in a planet of over 7 billion people, with roughly half of them being women, there will be a good number that find the bald pate either more attractive than hair or inconsequential to their decision on who to date.

Of course, there are other studies that show that women are 'biologically-wired' to choose men who have hair on their heads or some other such nonsense. If you ask me, that doesn't give women a lot of credit in making their own choices. To conclude that a woman can't make a conscious choice in whether or not she finds a man attractive, but instead gives into natural instinct, is kind of insulting.

6. It can be Age-defying

Pop quiz: Without looking it up on the Internet, how old are Bruce Willis, Samuel L. Jackson, Vin Diesel and Patrick Stewart? All of them are older than you think!

All of these men had adopted the bald by choice look years ago and have only benefitted from the fact that they don't have to worry about covering up grey hair or thinning spots. In many cases, these men can go 20 to 30 years with this look and it can be difficult for the public to see much change in them as they age.

Does that mean this will happen to you if you choose to shave off your hair? I can't promise you that, but I can assure you that if you adopt the look, take care of your health and walk around with good posture along with a smile on your face, you probably will appear a bit younger.

7. Rub Your Head for Luck...Anytime!

I don't know if you've ever experienced it before, but there's something truly liberating about rubbing your hand over your own scalp. It can be in the middle of a workday or just before going to bed. Feeling the skin on your hand against the short bristle or nearly bald scalp of your head is an invigorating experience. It's what being a man is all about.

We've covered some of the basics when it comes to some of the benefits to being bald. Next, we'll discuss how you could sabotage those advantages, if you're not careful.

The 8 Things to Avoid Doing as a Bald Man

The following are suggestions and points of discussion to consider. You already know where I stand in regards to the option to buzz or shave off your hair. However, you may be considering one or a few of the following. What I am about to share is a realistic assessment of some things to consider or not to consider if you are going to adopt this lifestyle:

1. Powders, Creams, Markers or any other Cover Up

Seriously, don't even bother with this stuff.

As I stated in the introduction, my intent in writing this book is to show you one way you can choose to live. That way is not by having to rub a smelly cream on your head or to spray weird chemicals on the scalp to create the appearance of hair. This also includes weird markers and cover up sprays that are marketed on late night infomercials or worse, on one of those home shopping channels.

You can say to yourself, 'Well, I will do it for a few more years and then when I become *too* bald, I'll stop and just buzz my hair off.'

I say, 'Why wait?'

All of the above 'solutions' are not only costly and time-consuming; they are also not always reliable. Further, they can become psychologically addictive. I know that sounds funny as you are not consuming any chemicals, but month after month, your scalp will begin to become more and more bare. When the time to shear your locks finally happens, you will likely end up where I did: covering almost as much of your head in a cover up powder as there is remaining hair on your head.

Not a way to live, my friend.

2. Toupees, Wigs or Transplants

Don't waste time with these. Honestly.

Toupees have now morphed into something called a 'hair system.' Still the same idea. Just some marketing genius using a thesaurus to prey on your insecurity. Regardless of what it's called, the result is still the same: Take a small pelt of artificial fur and glue it to the top of your head and then walk around thinking nobody knows you are wearing one.

If you are one of those people who currently is wearing a toupee, you'll have to forgive me for my boldness, but just stop doing it. You're not fooling anyone. I'm not trying to be cruel. My maternal grandfather wore a toupee for the last thirty years of his life. If anything, the mean people are the ones who are being nice to your face, but behind your back, they snicker to others about that ridiculous toupee. I mean, would it hurt for them to just tell you the truth?

Wigs fall into the same boat. The only two groups of people who should likely wear a wig from day-to-day are performers and those dealing with some sort of medical condition that has caused hair loss. For the latter, there is definitely the consideration that they haven't yet arrived psychologically or emotionally with the reality of their hair loss, especially children. As I have said before, those who have lost their hair from something other than the combination of the natural progression of aging and genetics are not the target readers of this book. However, I hope that some of them will come to see there is no shame in their losing their hair. Instead, it is my hope those individuals will see that there is more to them than the hair on their head or the wig they are wearing.

Finally, the hair transplant. I know, I know. They aren't called 'transplants' anymore. They're called 'hair reassignment,' 'hair stem cell relocation' or some other baloney. Again, marketing at work to prey on your insecurities!

Do I think these doctors should give up doing this for all of the gullible souls who choose to throw thousands of dollars at them to cut up their scalps and poke holes in the tops of their heads? No! It's a still a free market in western society and other parts of the world. If there are people willing to pay good sums of money to have this procedure done and go through the weeks of pain and recovery, then by all means, do it.

That being said, once the procedure is performed, shaving your skull or even buzzing your hair down to next to nothing may become an impossibility as you will be left with the telltale 'smiley' scar of the hair transplant on the back of your head. I know there are now procedures that tout 'no scars,' but I am skeptical myself about such claims and I think it would be wise if you were too.

The other thing I've noticed about hair transplants (and I've been around a few) is the balding that occurs behind the front of the transplanted hair. In other words, there is a potential problem with starting transplant procedures while there is still a decent amount of hair up top to create the illusion that nothing really ever changed. The problem is that after the hair is transplanted to the front, there is no guarantee it will take and if it does take, there's no guaranteed stoppage of hair falling out from behind the newly transplanted area. This means another procedure would have to be done after the first was performed a number of years later.[11]

Ask yourself: How many times am I willing to endure this costly and sometimes painful procedure?

3. Drugs or Lotions

I don't think I have to tell you that when you are taking a drug meant to do something like grow hair on top of your head that you wouldn't expect some side effects. Same goes for the 'regrowth' lotions and creams you are to rub on your head.

Do these things work? In most cases, success has been reported in growing back hair, but at what price?

Let's start with the pills. One of the leading sellers uses finasteride. The

---

[11] http://www.foxnews.com/health/2014/03/07/expert-warns-against-hair-transplants-for-men-in-their-20s/

manufacturer of these pills lists the following on their website as side effects:

- A decrease in sex drive
- Trouble getting or keeping an erection
- A decrease in the amount of semen
- Breast tenderness and enlargement along with lumps, pain or nipple discharge
- Depression
- A decrease in sex drive that can continue after stopping the medication
- An allergic reaction that includes rashes, itching, hives and swelling of the lips, tongue, throat, and face
- Problems with ejaculation that continue after stopping medication
- Testicular pain
- Difficulty in achieving an erection that continued after stopping the medication
- Male infertility and/or poor quality of semen
- In rare cases, male breast cancer.

They had my attention at 'a decrease in sex drive.'

The above are just some of the side effects taken from the manufacturer's *own* website.[12]

Is regrowing some or all of your hair back worth experiencing the numerous side effects from taking this drug? The above isn't meant to scare you into not doing it. However, be honest with yourself. When some side effect can last in your body well after you stop taking the drug, shouldn't that cause some alarm? We're talking about potentially permanent change here!

Okay, I've beaten the pill wagon to death. What about the topical solutions? Well, one of the leading solutions is minoxidil. Does it work? Just like the finasteride, it does work... in most cases. So you may be one of the many lucky souls who can rub this stuff on their scalp and watch as your hair follicles come to life all over again. But what are the side effects? Let's take a look:[13]

'Some people may experience a dry, itchy scalp and irritation.'

Actually, that's not too bad when you compare it to the last drug we reviewed.

---

[12]

https://www.merck.com/product/usa/pi_circulars/p/propecia/propecia_ppi.pdf

[13] http://www.rogaine.com/category/products/faqs.do

However, there are some other considerations for minoxidil. First, the same website for one of the leading manufacturers informs the potential buyer that their product is not to be stopped at any time or they will return back to the way things were before, therefore, you'll want to make their products 'part of your daily routine.'

If this is something that interests you and you are committed to doing it for the long haul, then maybe minoxidil is right for you. There are credible websites that have discussed the possibility of truly negative side effects of overdosing on the product. A quick Internet search can give you what you need.

4. Home Remedies

Yes, I was desperate enough for a short while that I purchased one of those 'bundles' of eBooks off of the Internet. This series of books recommended rubbing olive oil and rosemary on my scalp twice a day and wearing a shower cap around the house with a bunch of other household items to create this pasty gunk.

I don't know about you, but that does not sound like how I want to spend my free time. Not to mention, my kids would probably have had a field day watching dad wear salad dressing on his head with a shower cap around the house. If nothing else, I guess it would give them something to discuss in therapy when they're adults.

After reading some of the eBooks, I decided against trying out these home remedies, as it seemed like life was too short to be making salad dressing in my bathtub every night. Not to mention, there's the old standby question: 'If it really works, why don't the drug manufacturers or some other entity exploit it?'

Because it doesn't work.

5. Hairline Tattoos or Other Permanent Markings

In case you didn't know, this is really a thing!

If you suffer from alopecia or some other condition that really creates a noticeably odd hairline or uneven patches of bare scalp next to hair in odd places, this might be for you.

However, there are many concerns to consider when pondering this procedure:

- Are you prepared to maintain the shaved head look the rest of your life? Getting tattoo ink put into your skin means it will be permanent. If you want to grow back your hair, it might look especially funny when parts of your scalp are dark, but surrounded by much longer, lighter hair.

- Sometimes tattoo ink begins to turn blue. This can happen on the scalp.

- There is the possibility that parts of your hair will still fall out and the reapplication of new ink to those places could lead to an uneven look.

All of these things should be considerations before you decide to do this procedure. I think you'll know what I'm going to say. For me, I have some of the 'worst' balding possible with a patch of hair in the front, but it's my crown that is going bald. I don't worry about it though. I considered this procedure for about 5 minutes until I realized that if my goal were to shed some vanity by shedding my hair, this would set me back in my journey.

Also, I am aware that some of the celebrities featured earlier as case studies may have had this procedure done. This doesn't make it any more right for you. It was a personal choice on their part.

6. Scalp Massaging or Hanging Your Head off the Side of your Bed

This ties back to item 4. I remember my dad telling me that my paternal grandfather kept most of his hair because he hung his head over the side of his bed and would massage his scalp daily. I wonder if maybe my grandfather was just genetically blessed to keep most of his hair.

Anyway, this is again a use of your free time that you may want to be spending on a more worthwhile pursuit. As far as I understand it, there is no scientific evidence that it actually works.

7. Lots of side hair

For some guys, especially older men like Jack Welch, this is a look they cultivate. There are plenty of bald men who have the horseshoe shape around their craniums that have allowed the side and back hair to grow in on their heads. Personally, I think it makes some men look like clowns. I mean when you consider how many clowns are portrayed as bald on top with hair growing out of the sides and back, it's kind of a lot.

8. No Combovers! Ever!!!

If there's only one thing to take away from reading this book, it is this: Unless you are dressing up for Halloween, you are an undercover police officer or you are an actor taking on the role of a lifetime, do NOT attempt this.

I think the combover must creep up on most men to make them think it looks good. The top of your head starts to show more and more scalp. You might have some length in your hair and therefore, you think you can just grow a little more out on the side to comb it over to the side. One thing leads to another and then boom! You are now rocking a full-blown combover that will stand straight up in an opposing wind and will likely hang off the side of your head, completely exposing your bald spots when you kiss your mate in the morning. It's just not a good look. It never has been and it never will be.

Bonus Tip!

Those are the main things I think are linked back directly into your hair. However, if there is some new 'magic' product that requires a certain amount of time or money to maintain or avoid certain conditions like rain or wind, it's a waste of your time and money.

Not only that, it just reinforces your insecurity.

I also want to emphasize that there are certain practices that will not help the balding man such as an overly sedentary lifestyle combined with poor nutrition, but that's in the next chapter.

The 18 Actions to Take as a Bald Man

Here's the great news! One of the fastest ways to counter anxiety about something is to take action on it. Sometimes that means little actions; sometimes it means bigger actions. Regardless, when you are moving toward your goal and taking action to complete a task, your mind is engaged in something other than the thing you're worried about. It takes time, but you can definitely do it!

The following are a number of ideas to consider as you work on becoming the confident bald man I know you can be:

1. Develop Yourself From Within

I've mentioned it before, but it bears repeating. There have been other books and websites that are touting the same message I want to tell you: You are NOT your hair!

When you focus on your hair, you *can't* focus on the people and the world around you.

This also means more than just being good at something or some things like making lots of money or being able to perform an athletic skill really well.

Developing yourself from within means that you are overcoming your weaknesses and faults to become a better man. This means that if you're impatient and lose your temper, then you are working on developing more patience and self-control. If you have been caustic to others in professional and/or personal relationships, then it means you are trying to soften your edge toward them. If you make commitments, keep them, but don't make promises you know you'll break. It means loving more and hating less. Forgiving others when they've wronged you, but having the courage to stand up for yourself and for those who cannot stand up for themselves when the time is right.

Above all, it means developing a sense of humor. The Bald n Dashing man doesn't always have to be the funniest guy in the room, but he should be the one who takes himself the least seriously.

All of these things are a part of developing yourself into the positive force that you know you can become.

On top of that, how cool would it be to develop a greater understanding of the world around you? I don't just mean technology, but there's history, philosophy, science, literature, other cultures and so much more. The world awaits your engagement and if you choose to stop worrying about your hair, it becomes much more easy for you to engage with it.

2. Choose Worthy Bald Role Models

While this tip is a bit tongue in cheek, there can be some value to having a few other bald men to look up to. The Case Studies chapter will likely have given you some ideas that the Bald n Dashing look is being chosen by celebrities, athletes, leaders and others. Really, when it comes down to it, there are probably more positive role models in your personal life who may have adopted the Bald n Dashing look already.

However, what's more important than trying to emulate someone because of their hair, is trying to emulate someone because of how they actually are as a person.

3. Ease into the Cut

If you've never buzzed or shaved your head or haven't done it in many years, it may be shocking to you and those around you when you adopt this look. You should also consider that your skin tone might be different shades, as your hair would have naturally blocked the sun's rays out of some parts and caused you to have lighter patches of scalp. Be patient, as you may need the sun to color those parts of your skin.

The other consideration is to determine the sensitivity of the surface of your skin on your scalp. It could be very likely that if you went from having hair to putting a razor blade to your head, that you could cause folliculitis, which is an irritation of the hair follicles.[14] This is most often manifested with red bumps and clogged pores forming at the irritated site. If you do develop this condition, it is good to see a medical specialist, such as a dermatologist, to treat this since the condition can sometimes be viral or bacterial. This shouldn't be the reason to ultimately not shave your head. It is simply the reason to be smart about it.

If you have hair that is more than two or three inches in length, start with a buzz cut of a #3 guard or #4 guard on top with it cut shorter around the sides and back. You can progress from there a few weeks or months later with a #2 and then if you thought it was worth it, you could go to a #1.

If you choose to do things this way, it would be a good idea to see a stylist and have him or her perform the haircut. Just remember that during this transition phase,

---

[14] http://en.wikipedia.org/wiki/Folliculitis

you will have to maintain the look with more frequent haircuts. This may run counter to the whole 'fight vanity thing,' but know that eventually when you get it short enough, you will be able to just shave your own head whenever you like.

4. Get High Quality Hair Clippers

After you've 'eased into the cut,' it would be a good idea to invest in your own quality electric hair clippers. There are many brands out there so I'm not going to give an endorsement of one over the other. Just keep in mind a couple of things.

Make sure the guards you use on the clippers (if you choose to use a guard) are the same brand as the clippers you are using and that the guard fits perfectly. I purchased a guard that was one brand to put on my old hair clippers when I first buzzed my head. The guard fell off a few times and left me with shorter patches than everywhere else. Finally I just caved and picked up a nice, affordable electric clippers kit that was specifically designed for balding men. Since that time, I no longer use a guard and I love it!

I'm not going to give instructions on how to go about buzzing your hair, but instead will direct you to at least website by following the footnote here[15]. Not to get too technical, but this webpage will refer to the activity as 'shaving' your head when in reality, it is more like giving your head a really close buzz cut.

The nice advantage to buzzing your head over shaving it is that you can get away with cutting your hair a bit less frequently than when you shave your scalp and the 5 o'clock shadow appears within a day or so.

5. Get a High Quality Razor

If you choose to shave the hair off down to your scalp, this will require a slightly different approach. If you do choose to go the route of the razor and I think it is worth consideration, here are a few really great sites to get you started on the process of shaving your head:

http://menshair.about.com/od/malecelebrit yhairstyles/a/headshave.htm

http://www.headshaver.org/how-to-shave-your-head/

Here is another site that talks about some of your other options:

http://www.baldrus.com/archives/what-is-the-best-way-to-shave-your-head/

---

[15]http://www.wikihow.com/Shave-Your-Head

6. Take Your Head and Face Shape into Account

Thank goodness we all don't look exactly alike! Some of us have heads that are more round while others might have heads that are broader, giving them an almost cube-like appearance. Some men have prominent chins and small noses while other men have the opposite. Regardless of what your head and face shape look like, remember that its okay to play around with the look a little bit.

You are not obligated to adopt one look and then stick with it the rest of your life. If you want to try growing out your hair a la Jason Statham at some point to hide a scar or cover some bumps on your head and add some accessories to your look like a big clunky watch or some glasses, go for it! If you want to grow some sort of facial hair or let the hair grow out an extra week or so, go for it. There are no hard and fast rules to the Bald n Dashing look! The key is to be confident in yourself as a man and not put your confidence in how you look.

7. Some Facial Hair Might be a Good Thing

Goatees, beards and mustaches in all of their shapes and sizes are still an option for you. Some men instinctively grow some facial hair once they shave their heads. It might be a way of offsetting the fact there is no hair on top of the head thus drawing the eyes downward or it could be more simply that the man in question thought it would enhance their 'cool' factor. Whatever the case, go ahead and experiment with different looks. You never know when you'll stumble across something that works.

In my case, after I buzzed my hair, I kept a clean-shaven look for about 6 months. There came a point when I decided to just allow a few days facial hair to come in and then trim it into a very short beard. The best part? The creation of this new look has led to more compliments that I look like I'd lost weight and look fitter than when I was still growing hair or was completely clean shaven.

8. Eyebrow, Nose and Ear Hair Control

If you don't already have one, invest in a quality hair trimmer for your eyebrows, nose and ears. It seems kind of silly to spend all this time taking hair off of the top of your head, but letting a uni-brow grow or having long straggly hairs hanging out of your ears. When you're mindful of these problem areas, it gets easier and easier to take care of them.

9. Wash Your Face & Scalp

Like any other person on Earth, you will probably be subject to skin problems. You will get acne from time-to-time and you may develop bumps or a rash. The trick is to minimize this as much as possible.

Now that you have an exposed scalp, treat it similar to how you treat your face: with care. If you weren't washing your face much before, then follow the same routine. However, if you do notice breakouts here and there, consider a facial washing routine that would include taking care of the bare parts of your scalp. In extreme cases, it would be a good idea to speak with your dermatologist.

10. Smell Good

I know you're probably thinking, "Really? This is an important tip?"

Of course! Attracting women and interacting with people in general for business or pleasure is more than just how you look and what you say. It's also about the nonverbal cues you send off and that includes the way you smell.

Bathe daily, wear deodorant and wear a subtle, but pleasing cologne. If you're having trouble choosing a scent, try taking a woman you trust with you to pick one out.

11. Have Confidence in Your Facial and other Features

Every person has some attractive attribute. I know you may have a hard time believing me as you go through this process of hair loss and ultimately choose to become Bald n Dashing. However, it's true.

We can't all be blessed to look like Chris Hemsworth, Blair Underwood or Antonio Banderas, but why should that even be a concern? Maybe you were blessed with broad shoulders and a nice smile. Be confident in those things. It could be that you have nice eyes, a deep voice and you're much taller than the average person. Embrace those qualities.

It's about being confident in who you are and what outwardly makes you unique.

I'll give a personal example. Since buzzing my head, I get more complements on my eyes and voice than I ever got when I still had the hair. Coincidence? Maybe. I'd like to think that one less distraction (my hair) is now what has led to people noticing some of my other qualities.

12. Wear Hats and Accessorize from Time-to-Time

Some men who choose to go bald by choice can really benefit from wearing a hat. It doesn't just have to be a baseball cap. Sometimes a stylish flat cap or fedora with a funky design might be your thing. If you weren't wearing a lot of hats prior to shaving off your hair, this might be a good time to give it a try. You never have to worry about messing up your hair.

It just makes sense to wear a hat when you are out in the sun for more than a few minutes. Where I live, almost every day is sunshine. There is rarely a cloudy day. The scalp needs to be protected, which leads me to my next point.

13. Get a Good Sunscreen for the Face

Skin cancer runs in my family. It might or might not run in yours, but why find out the hard way? Wearing sunscreen on a regular basis will prevent this.

Men who are fair-skinned will definitely need to be aware of this. I have rather fair skin and I have learned that being out in the southwest desert for more than a few minutes without sunscreen can lead to a pink scalp, which is the beginning of sunburn.

There are many products on the market and it is up to you to choose what is best. I have tried different products and have found many to work quite well. I would only emphasize that you look for something specifically made to protect the face. Other sunscreens for the body may be oilier than the ones for the face. This can create a 'slick' appearance on the face and also could lead to clogged pores for some people.

When applying the sunscreen for your face and scalp, be sure to apply it evenly and not to miss too many spots. It is also good to apply to the ears and back of the neck as these areas are now fully exposed.

You may be worried that the coloring of your scalp will be uneven without unimpeded sun exposure. This is just a part of the transition process. It will likely only last for a few weeks and then your scalp will look much more even and natural.

14. Wear Stylish Clothes

You don't need to go out and drop thousands of dollars to overhaul your wardrobe. However, take an assessment of what you currently own and whether or not it is currently in style. If you're making a life transition to no hair, this is a perfect time to adopt some new styles into your wardrobe.

Maybe you were wearing baggy jeans before you shaved your head, but you can get away with slim fit. Go buy a pair and see what happens. It could be that you were a T-shirt guy, but now polo shirts seem to go with your look better. Have you ever tried tailored fit, fitted or slim fit shirts? If you have the physique to pull it off, but have been hesitant, wait no longer. Now is the time.

Embrace it! That leads me to the next point.

15. Wear Collared Shirts

In the Bald n Dashing lifestyle, there should be very few hard and fast rules. This idea is more of an option for consideration, but most men who are bald by choice may not have the most defined jaw lines. Wearing a shirt that has a downward angle to the collar may be the very thing that creates the illusion of a more defined jaw line.

The regular crew neck T-shirt, while useful for exercising and wearing as a layer under another collared shirt, has a shape to the neckline that really does not enhance a balding man's features. The v-shape that a collared shirt provides can do it much better.

16. Get into and Stay in Decent Shape

Do you have six-pack abs? Neither do I. It's okay though. The other day, I just read an interview with a famous Hollywood actor who is giving up the role of a superhero he's portrayed for a long-time because he's sick of the super-strict diet that leads him to look super lean and super awesome.

Realistically, most of us will never look like a superhero or a professional athlete. Those who have achieved that look and functionality do so with amazing social, mental, emotional and physical discipline. There are even fewer of those people who will be able to maintain that state for years, if not decades to come.

That isn't my goal. What is my goal is to have a functional, healthy-looking body that is capable of not only performing basic physical tasks that don't completely toll the body. Being able to lift more than a 135 pounds over my head repeatedly or running for more than just a few minutes without being winded are really the kinds of goals I focus on when I workout. However, you may be in much better shape than that. If that's the case, just continue to look for ways to improve. Not everyone is going to be genetically blessed with big arms and a tiny waist any more than being blessed with a full head of hair.

The main thing I want you to take away from this point is to eat well, stay away from fad diets, drugs and exercise programs and maintain regular fitness. You will not transform overnight, but as you progress from day to day, setting and meeting smaller goals to get to bigger ones, you will begin to transform into that fitter, healthier you.

17. Laugh at Hair Transplant Advertisements

This might be one of the most important actions you can take as a bald man.

Remember, these hair transplant ads are designed specifically to make you feel insecure and unwanted. That's the whole point of marketing, right?

After you've buzzed or shaved off your hair, I would like to suggest the following exercise. The next time you see an advertisement for one of these hair restoration 'institutes,' you should laugh and point at the screen. It doesn't matter if you're home alone, at the bar with some friends or sitting on the couch with your girlfriend. Point and laugh.

Now, before you think I'm recommending you act like someone who belongs in a looney bin, let me explain. Men who are Bald n Dashing need to have a sense of humor. You are not necessarily laughing at the actors portrayed as insecure in the commercial and you're not laughing at the actors in the lab coats who are portraying the doctors. You're laughing at this concept: That you are not a complete man because you are going bald. By laughing out loud and having a little fun with the whole thing, you are reminding yourself not to take all of this so seriously.

You are Bald n Dashing and a Bald n Dashing man should have a sense of humor!

18. Shine a Spotlight on It

Okay, we all know the jokes about baldheads and reflective light.

Moving on.

There is a nautical term that is used for dealing with a negative event or potentially difficult situation. It's called 'sailing into the wind.[16]'

When a sailing crew wants to head in the direction that the wind is coming from, there is no way to angle the sail directly against the wind and move forward. Instead, the boat and its sail will take an angled approach to utilize the wind's force and still head in the general direction the crew wants to go.

[16] http://en.wikipedia.org/wiki/Sailing_into_the_wind

How does this help you?

The simple answer is that just like the sailors realized they couldn't take the opposing force of the wind on directly, they choose to use their brains and creativity to solve the problem. That's what I am hoping for you.

Which brings us full circle from action number 1 at the beginning of this chapter.

Develop a sense of humor or use the one you've already got.

When you first shave or buzz your head, you are going to encounter some jokes from time to time. That's okay. Let the jokes come. You may even notice more jokes to your face than the jokes others might have said behind your back when you were trying to hide the thinning hair. If this is the case, take it as a compliment, because it means that you appear confident enough to take it.

The thing to keep in mind is that it doesn't hurt to have a few jokes of your own ready to go. It certainly does you no good to take other people's jokes or even insults to heart. If anything, it will just make the problems worse.

Being able to give a few off-the-cuff humorous and sometimes self-deprecating remarks from time to time is a major positive. It can be disarming and in many cases, cause people to take a deeper interest in you.

I'll share a few of brief examples:

I was meeting with some clients who had mistakenly thought I was one of my business partners. I corrected them and then let them know if I was that particular business partner, I would be a lot taller and I would have a full head of hair, but I wouldn't be as good looking. The clients laughed and the tone was set for a cooperative, light-hearted meeting.

Another time, I had a friend who was ribbing me for losing my hair while he still has a full head of hair. After a couple of light-hearted jibes, I simply said 'You know, I feel bad for you. Not all of us can have the problem condition called *testosteronus elevatum*.' He got the joke and his jokes slowed down. The point wasn't that I really had higher testosterone than him, but rather that if the light-hearted ribbing was going to continue; it was going to be returned in kind.

Finally, I remember volunteering at a school a while back and a student asked me why I was bald. I told him that some of my favorite action stars were men who'd shaved their heads and I thought it looked cool. He seemed to like that answer.

Don't put yourself down brutally in other people's eyes, but rather to show you are fully aware that you are going bald and that you made the active choice to break up with your hair before it broke up with you.

Hopefully, you found the suggested actions useful. Take which ones you like and adopt them and keep the others on reserve, just in case. None of this is all encompassing. Instead, these are ideas and primers to help you get on with your life and make things as easy as possible as you transition into the Bald n Dashing lifestyle.

Bald by Choice

If you are choosing to make the change after reading some or all parts of this book, congratulations! You are on your way to a whole new world of possibilities and potential!

Remember that if you are choosing to shave or buzz your hair off is that this is *your* choice. I know it wasn't your choice to lose your hair and it wasn't your choice on how society has treated you because of it, but it is your choice to do something about it now and if shaving it all off is what you've chosen, then the choice has definitely been yours!

Remember, not everyone is going to embrace your new look. However, that's not up to you. You are not responsible for other people's feelings. You are responsible for yourself and how you feel. It may take a little time, but most people who react in a less than positive manner to the shaved head usually come around and sometimes even become fans.

The time has come to own this new choice!

Own It!

When I set out to write this book, I didn't think it would be so much fun! I really have enjoyed the process of sharing with you the many ideas and tips I've picked up over the years as I've adopted the bald by choice lifestyle. Am I really Bald n Dashing? You know, some days I feel like I am! However, I go through trials and stress like everyone else and I can feel down about some circumstances that arise from time to time.

But the most important thing that I remember is that I am more than my hair. As I said at the beginning, there really is <u>no</u> shame in going bald. It should never even be considered a failure. You are not the hair that sits on your head. You never were and you never will be.

I really hope something shared in these pages made an impact on you. There are many men out there who feel insecure and a bit hopeless about going bald. My message has been and always will be to stop worrying about it, take action and move on to the much more important, meaningful and ultimately satisfying parts of life. Your life is too short and so is mine. That means it is probably time for me to end this book.

But before I go, I want to share with you one of my favorite poems. I first read it when I was 16 years old. Decades later, it means so much more to me. As you read it, you will see the underlying theme that has permeated the entire Bald n Dashing lifestyle:

If

If you can keep your head when all about you

Are losing theirs and blaming it on you,

If you can trust yourself when all men doubt you,

But make allowance for their doubting too;

If you can wait and not be tired by waiting,

Or being lied about, don't deal in lies,

Or being hated, don't give way to hating,

And yet don't look too good, nor talk too wise:

If you can dream—and not make dreams your master;

If you can think—and not make thoughts your aim;

If you can meet with Triumph and Disaster

And treat those two impostors just the same;

If you can bear to hear the truth you've spoken

Twisted by knaves to make a trap for fools,

Or watch the things you gave your life to, broken,

And stoop and build 'em up with worn-out tools:

If you can make one heap of all your winnings

And risk it on one turn of pitch-and-toss,

And lose, and start again at your beginnings

And never breathe a word about your loss;

If you can force your heart and nerve and sinew

To serve your turn long after they are gone,

And so hold on when there is nothing in you

Except the Will which says to them: "Hold on!"

If you can talk with crowds and keep your virtue,

Or walk with Kings—nor lose the common touch,

If neither foes nor loving friends can hurt you,

If all men count with you, but none too much;

If you can fill the unforgiving minute

With sixty seconds' worth of distance run,

Yours is the Earth and everything that's in it,

And—which is more—you'll be a Man, my son.[17]

Now go out there and be the man you're supposed to be! Take care of the hair, take care of yourself, your family, and your friends and be Bald n Dashing!

_____

[17] http://en.wikisource.org/wiki/If—

Other Resources

While making my decision to buzz all of my hair off my head, I did what any other guy would do and scoured the Internet for emotional support and validation. Okay, not every guy does this, but I did find some of the following resources helpful as I made the decision to take off my hair.

Check them out:

1. **Sly Bald Guys** - www.slybaldguys.com - This is a great support community that boasts more than 10 000 members! If you're struggling with the ability to get past the fact you are losing your hair, give this website your full attention. When I was considering the buzz cut that would change my life, this site was a major resource.

2. **Bald R Us** - www.baldrus.com - Founded by bald man Tony Snesko, Bald R Us is a website that gives many great ideas and links to communities that can help you regain your confidence and become the powerful force you know you were always meant to be.

3. **Slick Bald Guys** - www.slickbaldguys.com - This is another website that appears to be in development,

but has some great instructions on shaving your head.

The following websites sell products that specialize in helping bald men achieve a certain look. I have not used every product on the websites, so I cannot endorse them. However, it may be wise to check them out as they have developed followings of their own:

1. **The HeadBlade** - www.headblade.com - I remember when I first saw this product a couple years after its debut in 1997. I was just about to go back into college and with the knowledge that I was losing my hair, I flirted with the idea of shaving it all off at that time. I chickened out at that time and I've chosen to buzz my hair instead of blade it, but I can definitely tell you that I have been very impressed with what they have to offer, including their premiere product, the HeadBlade. Great stuff.

2. **Bee Bald** - www.beebald.com - With lots of great scrubs and lotions, this site is worth a gander. This company has developed products that not only work for men who are balding or bald by choice, these products are great for people who have sensitive skin.

Anyway, I hope you find what you're looking for with some of these websites. Every day, more and more men are making the choice to be bald and it is likely that more sites like these will spring up. Check them out.

An Invitation

Like the book? I'd love a review!

Your positive feedback on www.Amazon.com helps other readers know what you thought about this book.

Also from publisher Paul St. George Press and this author: 'The Great Big Love Quote Book,' 'The Great Big Fitness Quote Book' and 'The Great Big Success Quote Book' are all on sale at Amazon.com.

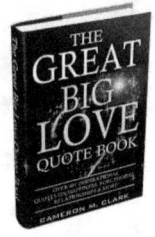 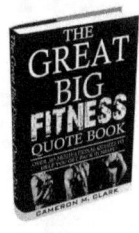 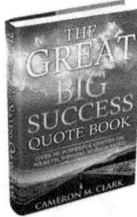

Thanks again for reading!

About the Author

Cameron M. Clark is a business development manager and former partner in a locally owned professional services company in Las Vegas, Nevada. He holds a Bachelors of Science in Communications from Southern Utah University. He and his wife, Cara are the parents of three children.